The En

A DO-IT-YOURSELF GUIDE TO OVERCOMING FATIGUE AND RESTORING ENERGY

Qiang Chen

Copyright © 2016 by Qiang Chen
All Rights Reserved

PREFACE

I believe the most profound ideas are always taught more effectively by simple language.

Many of the ideas in this book originate from my grandma. She didn't go to school. The only Chinese characters she could write was her name. When I was a young boy growing up in a small tea-planting village near Hangzhou, China, I always heard her nagging at her grandchildren about covering up the belly button to prevent an upset stomach, drinking ginger tea to warm up the body after getting wet in the rain and so on. Years later during my study at the Chinese Medical University, I found that many Chinese medical teachings on healthy living were similar to my granny's advice- only she explained things in simple day-to-day language that made more sense.

I try to use the same simple language to outline my thoughts on restoring energy and wellbeing in this book.

Many of us are living fast paced, stressful lives and facing fatigue, burn out and poor health as a result. Although it is good to see more people in the West turning to natural and holistic methods such as acupuncture to recharge and fix health issues; the treatment and advice that Chinese medicine doctors offer is normally not understood and hard to follow.

This book provides an easy to understand and use tool set for restoring energy and vitality, based on the insights I've gained from over two decades of practicing Chinese Medicine.

ACKNOWLEDGMENT

Thanks to my wife, Shuang and our son Harry, for their endless support and encouragement despite the time that writing this book took me away from them. Thanks also to Farzad Sharifi-Yazdi for editing: without his passion, deep understanding of the subject and language skills this book would never have its easy to read and smooth flow. Above all I want to thank all the people who trust me and allow me to support their journey in recovery.

TABLE OF CONTENTS

PREFACE	3
Acknowledgement	5
Table of Contents	7
INTRODUCTION	9
Chapter 1. Sleeping Well	25
Chapter 2. Eat and Digest Well	33
Chapter 3. Exercise Well	45
Chapter 4. Emotional Wellbeing	53
CLOSING REMARKS	61
Appendix 1. Guide to Choosing an Acupuncturist.	63
Appendix 2. Separation & Detachment	67
Appendix 3. Acceptance	69
Appendix 4: Anger and Fear Release	71
Appendix 5: Cultivate Positive Emotions	73
About The Author	75

INTRODUCTION

Why You Should Read This Book

Have you recently experienced any of the following conditions?

* Waking up feeling tired, no matter how long you have slept.

* Overactive mind: unable to switch off at bedtime.

* Poor appetite in the morning and noon (skipping meals); cravings and overeating in late afternoons and evenings.

* Feeling bloated, fatigued and with sugar craving after meals.

* Irregular and poorly formed bowel movement: feeling drained or still feel not empty after the job is done.

* Cold hands and feet - even in the summer time.

* Mood swings and not at peace with your own company.

* Low or no libido.

* Getting sick more frequently and experiencing long recovery times.

If your answer to any of the above is yes, this book is for you.

An analogy I like to use is that maintaining optimal health is like caring for a car. If you have a range of discomforts but have had no illness identified by doctors - it is like a car that is still drive-able but worn down (e.g. oil leak and low battery) and in need of a tune up.

In Chinese medicine, the symptoms listed on previous page are considered as red lights on the body's dashboard. Each 'red light' or symptom has its underlying indication;

*** Fatigue in the morning:** means the body is unable to recharge its battery (energy) effectively through sleep.

* **Unable to switch off at bedtime**: means the racing mind has built up too much momentum throughout the day - and so slowing down by night time has become too hard or takes too long.

* **Lacking appetite in the morning**: means a weak or overloaded digestive tract has failed to empty on time and therefore not rested and recovered by the morning.

* **Bloating and fatigue after meals**: means the stomach is weak and lacks the sufficient blood flow for digestion after meals so it borrows the blood supply from the brain and muscles - leading to a foggy mind and physical tiredness. The bloating shows that energy absorbed from the digestive tract has not been distributed efficiently and is trapped in the abdominal region.

* **Sugar cravings:** means the body is low on energy because a weak digestive system is not converting food into sugar efficiently. To compensate, the body is looking for an immediate sugar boost.

* **Irregular and poorly formed bowel movement**: means that the large intestine is sluggish and unable to eliminate garbage effectively.

* **Cold hands and feet:** means poor blood circulation in the limbs as a result of energy depletion. In this situation, the body reduces blood supply to less important areas such as the digestive tract, hands and feet in order to safeguard supply to critical organs such as the brain and heart.

* **Experiencing mood swings**: means that you are low on energy and facing a regular outpouring of repressed emotions.

* **Low or no libido**: means the body's energy levels are so low that it has to cut down energy supply to less urgent systems such as the reproductive system.

* **Getting sick easily and difficulty recuperating**: means the body is weak and low on immunity and also lacking the energy to repair and recover properly.

You may notice that almost all of the above symptoms are rooted in low energy and fatigue. Intuitively, we try to fix the surface layer signs of fatigue without seeing what is beneath it. So people drink coffee or caffeine-rich energy drinks to seek an instant energy boost. Many self-help books encourage readers to be hyper-focused on man-made goals and to push through physical warning signs and emotional lows.

People also shop around in supplement stores and natural therapy clinics trying to get a quick fix for their exhaustion. But, as soon as their symptoms are relieved, they resume the same lifestyle that led to an energy depletion in the first place. It is as though the driver has acknowledged a red light on the dashboard, pulled over and simply placed a band-aid over the red light and resumed driving. The red light is an important and helpful warning. If the driver ignores it and maintains an abusive driving pattern, the car is destined to break down quickly and permanently.

The right way to address fatigue at its core and fix it for the long term, is to lead a lifestyle in which you are recharging more energy than you are using up. In doing this it can be useful to look at this from the perspective of Chinese Medicine.

The Three Energy Levels & 5 Stages of Human Health

According to the Chinese, overall health and wellbeing is governed by three levels of energy called the 'three treasures': *Jing*, *Qi*, and *Shen*.

Jing is inherent energy reserves we are born with and is largely determined by genetics. So each person has different levels of this reserve energy, but it is a limited resource that will end at some point - when we die of natural causes. However, a healthy lifestyle can help to replenish and prolong this reserve. For example, good sleep is one way in which it can be boosted.

Qi (pronounced Chee) is the inherent life force and energy in all things and flows through and animates the movement of our body. It is cultivated mainly from the air we inhale and food that is properly digested.

Shen is effectively the energy of our spirit and higher consciousness - and thus where the sense of peace and purpose in our life can flow from. If the Chi and Jing are well preserved, then our Shen tends to be strong and balanced too.

It's not necessary to go further in the details of these ideas here, you can find many good books and online resources for this. However, the underlying principles of the 'three treasures' or what I call the 'three energies' are important to the discussion on fatigue- so I'll use them in the following simplified form:

1) Jing: inherent **reserve energy** of body.

2) Qi: **actual energy** activating the body.

3) Shen: **emotional & spiritual energy**

As a Chinese Medicine practitioner these three energy levels form the lens through which I view fatigue and energy recharge. We can understand how they work and effect our health by using the '**5 Stages of Human Health***' Table over the page.

* Inspired by Qingzhong Wu, "Ren Ti Shi Yong Shou Ce (*The User's Manual for Human Body*)" Chinese Edition 2005.

Table 1: Five Stages of Human Health*

Health State	STAGE 1 HEALTHY	STAGE 2 LOW IMMUNITY	STAGE 3 SUPERMAN	STAGE 4 FATIGUED	STAGE 5 EXHAUSTED (Disease)
Energy Levels	- High Energy - Reserve energy untouched	- Low Energy - Reserve energy largely unused	- Energy half full - Reserved energy in greater use	- Energy very low - Reserved energy low	- Energy critically low - Reserved energy very low
Signs	- Sleep well - Eating well - Emotional balance - Healthy libido	- Mildly fatigued - Susceptible to colds, flu & headaches	- 'Invincible' mindset - 'Night Owl' - Hotel Room Syndrome	- Frequent Fatigue - Mood swings - Short energy surges & sudden lows	- Constant fatigue - Emotionally low - Susceptible to chronic & systematic diseases.
Energy Chart					

Let us look at these five stages of human health shown in the table in more detail.

In Stage 1 we are at the optimal level of health; we are full of energy and so our reserve energy remains untouched and well preserved. Our sleep is good, we enjoy a balanced diet and good digestion and bowel movement; we also exercise well and feel emotionally stable and well-balanced.

However, if we push ourselves hard and fail to recharge regularly through good sleep, diet, and restorative exercises and mental relaxation, we will fall into Stage 2.

In Stage 2 we are mildly fatigued or what I call '**Low Immunity State**'. Our body has less energy - but our reserve energy remains largely unused. As we have lower energy we are more susceptible to minor ailments like colds, flu and headaches. If we do not recharge properly through the right means, we enter Stage 3.

In Stage 3 our energy levels fall just below half full. However, as we keep pushing our body forward at full pace, our reserve energy is put into greater use. This gives us an energy surge, and temporary feeling of invincibility; so we do more than we are normally capable of, which is why I also call this stage the **Superman State**. I've seen many businessmen, entrepreneurs, hyper driven students and even some mothers fall into this category.

Tell-tale signs of people in this stage include: the need to be constantly occupied with something and unable to sit still, night owls whose brain activity peaks in the late hours and, what I call the 'hotel room syndrome' where as soon as you reach the holiday hotel room you are hit by a nasty cold or flu - which is your body's attempt to use the downtime to fix and recharge itself. But people at this stage often repress the natural healing process with strong medication in order to get back to full activity as soon as possible.

And rather than restore energy through good sleep, diet, exercise and so on - the false sense of invincibility often leads to more destructive patterns i.e. late nights, over eating, high intake of fast and processed/junk food, high alcohol intake and no exercise or fanatic in extreme sports that further depletes the reserve energy.

Sooner or later this all takes its toll as the body runs even shorter on energy and reserve energy and enters Stage 4. Remember, reserve '*Jing*' energy is largely genetic, so some may have more of it than others; but, it is also a limited resource so will ultimately run out if you persistently fail to rest and recharge whilst leading such a full-on lifestyle.

In Stage 4 our energy and our reserve energy are both running low and we are physically fatigued much of the time. We may have momentary surges in energy if we push ourselves using our reserve energy but these short surges are followed by a sudden low. These highs and lows are matched with mood swings.

More prolonged and serious illnesses that are harder to recover from may also start to arise and persist in this stage. If we fail to see these physical and emotional warning signs and continue to drive on without stopping for a substantial recharge we will reach stage 5.

In Stage 5 our energy is at emergency low levels and our reserve energy is also running extremely low. We are fatigued and emotionally low and are susceptible to chronic and systematic diseases (a weak body and negative emotions provide a fertile breeding ground for disease). Recovering from this stage and it associated diseases becomes an uphill struggle as we are low on the reserve energy that is designed primarily to help us fight such emergency problems. Medical intervention is usually required in this stage.

How to Recharge and Restore Vitality

Sadly, many people these days are mildly to seriously fatigued and so stuck somewhere between Stages 2 to 4. In-fact, the majority of the patients that came to see me are in Stage 4. The problem with this state is that there is often no identifiable 'problem' for conventional doctors to deal with. So most of the signs I've described are either ignored or put down to stress and, most people are not clear what practical steps to take to overcome it.

Our most urgent aim must therefore be rise out of Stages 2 to 4, avoid Stage 5 and return to and remain in

Stage 1! So how can we do this and ensure that we are always enjoying optimal health? We can begin by asking ourselves 4 simple questions that are universally applicable and understood:

* Are you sleeping well?

* Are you eating and pooing well?

* Are you exercising well?

* Are you feeling at peace?

These questions can form a simple four pillar approach to recharging and restoring vitality.

The Four Pillars of Energy Recharge

Below are what I consider to be the '4 pillars' or signs of optimal health (i.e. Stage 1):

1. **Sleeping well**: waking up feeling refreshed and having adequate energy for the entire day.

2. **Eating & digesting well**: feeling hungry at mealtimes, satisfied with meals without fatigue and bloating.

Passing formed stool at least once a day and feeling light afterwards.

3. **Exercising well**: feeling warm and energized after exercises that promote good breathing and movement.

4. **Emotional wellbeing**: feeling in control and at peace with yourself, your emotions and your life.

The following four chapters offer a simple step by step guide on what you can do in each of these four areas to restore your energy and wellbeing. Consider this pocket book as your do-it-yourself manual for rebooting and recharging your body!

Acupuncture as a Complimentary Tool

You will find that at the end of each chapter I offer a snapshot of my insights on how acupuncture also helps with: sleeping well, eating and digesting well, exercising well and emotional wellbeing. I focus on acupuncture as a tool specifically because that is my expertise and I have personally seen its great benefits and results for the countless fatigued and unwell patients I have treated over the past two decades.

In very simple terms - acupuncture works in the same way as pressing the "Ctrl" "Alt" and "Del" on your computer, resetting and rebooting the body's blocked energy system. This allows the body's natural healing mechanisms to effectively do its work on restoring your overall energy levels and wellbeing.

So I encourage you to do some research and give it a go to confirm my claim for yourself (See Appendix 1 for my simple guide to choosing the right acupuncturist). But do not forget that I'm recommending acupuncture as an additional tool to compliment the practical steps offered in the following pages.

Chapter 1. Sleeping Well

Sleeping is without doubt the most important part of recharging. A simple way to check if you are sleeping well is to ask yourself if you feel rested when you open your eyes in the morning.

Over the years, I've heard many answers to this question:

* I keep pushing the snooze button on my alarm clock until it is absolutely the last minute.

* I drag myself out of bed, only feeling better after a shower and strong coffee.

* I am not a morning person. It takes a few hours or the entire morning to be fully awake.

* I just get out of bed and start my day, no matter how my body feels.

* My energy, if it not at zero, is in minus in the mornings.

These are sadly very common statements that many people relate to but it needn't be this way. Here are some steps you can take to ensure better recharge from sleep:

1. Sleep at the right hours

As often as possible try to be in deep sleep by 11pm. Why? Because humans, like many other animals have built-in biological clocks that keep the body in step with the rising and setting of the sun. The ancient Chinese noticed our body's energy (*Qi*) flows through meridians in a well-defined rhythm, in which the maximum energy levels flowed through different meridians at different times in the 24-hour circle. Chinese believe that the best time for energy recharge is between the 'golden hours' of 11pm to 3am, when maximum energy flows through the gallbladder and liver meridians - both of which are involved in the detoxification of the whole body. These are therefore the most effective hours for restoring digestive energy and detoxifying and so the time that you should be in deep sleep in order to allow this work to take place. This echoes with the old English saying 'every hour spent asleep before midnight is worth two hours after midnight'.

2. Adopt Healthy Pre-Sleep Habits

What you do in the hours just before going to bed can have a big impact on how quickly you fall asleep and the quality of your sleep. Here are 3 steps you can easily adopt for a better sleep; the first two are tried and tested habits in Chinese culture:

a) Eat early or eat light in the evening and go to bed with an empty stomach. If you go to bed with a full stomach, your body is not resting or detoxing but working hard on digesting food.

b) Take a hot foot bath before bed. Specifically, you can soak your feet in a bucket of warm water, making sure to submerge them two inches above the ankle bone and keep them soaking for fifteen minutes or more until your forehead is clammy. This pre-sleep foot bath ensures that more blood goes to the feet and legs and less to the head allowing the mind to slow down and feel more relaxed as you go to bed.

c) Keep all communication and entertainment devices out of the bedroom. If the mind is constantly engaged with information, it takes time to unwind. Just like the momentum of a fast turning wheel, it takes longer to slow down. Let your bedroom be your sacred space, for resting and energy recharge only. Leave entertainment (including TV, laptops, tablets and smart phones) out of your bedroom. More importantly refrain from using these devices for at least the one hour before going to bed. For those that need to use their phone as an alarm clock, you can leave it outside the bedroom - so that you have to physically get out of bed to switch it off in the morning.

3. Sleep well throughout the night

If you follow the first two steps well, it is more than likely that you will enjoy a long and uninterrupted sleep throughout the night. However, there may be times that -for whatever reason- we wake up at odd hours in the night. In most cases when this happens, people toss and turn, stressed about not being able to fall back to sleep.

The trick I have learned from one of my patients is to not stress about it. Indeed, when she wakes up in the middle of the night, she will say, "good, I have extra time to do my meditation." She will then lie in bed as comfortably as she can, being mindful of her breathing, and watching her thoughts wander. Once she does that, she usually starts to relax and slip back to sleep. If she is unable to go back to sleep after an hour, she keeps reminding herself, "even if I haven't slept, I am resting. I will be okay to function in the morning."

This is great advice which you can use when necessary, keeping in mind to accept the situation and to not stress about it as that would just make matters worse.

4. Take Regular Power Naps

If for any reason you feel drowsy during the day - especially for shift workers or new parents who have been deprived of good sleep- an effective tool for quickly recharging during the daytime can be a short power nap. Napping is in fact a very common custom in some countries including China, Japan and of some Mediterranean countries.

For example, a nap after lunch was part of the school curriculum I grew up with in China, and it was practiced throughout my primary to high school. Today many factory workers in China are given a short break for napping after lunch.

In the last decade, many researchers have confirmed that napping is both physiologically and psychologically beneficial. Here is how you can maximize the benefit of it:

* A power nap should not exceed twenty minutes; otherwise you slip into a deep sleep mode and wake up feeling groggy.

* It works best between one and three p.m., according to the natural pattern of our body clock.

* Avoid napping after work or after five p.m., which may interrupt your sleep at night.

* If you are unable to switch off your mind easily, try a five-minute 'guided meditation' break. It is equally powerful and effective. Download a meditation app on your phone, plug in an earphone, and enjoy. Personally,

I use a wonderful app called 'Insight Timer' which you can download from https://insighttimer.com.

Acupuncture for Sleeping Well

Over the years nearly all patients I've seen for a wide range of issues report of better sleep after treatment. This is probably down to:

* Releases of endorphins (body's natural painkiller) during acupuncture.

* Release of Serotonin (body's natural happy chemical) during acupuncture.

* Above chemicals relieve a restless mind & tense body allowing you to relax and sleep.

Chapter 2. Eat and Digest Well

Eat and digest well consists of external and internal components: the food we eat is the external aspect and how well this food is absorbed and eliminated from the body is the internal aspect.

Most people focus on the external part of eating - i.e. diet plans and food choices (Organic vs GMO); there are plenty of good books and online resources out there on this topic. From a Chinese medicine perspective however, greater emphasis is placed on the internal aspect of eating and therefore the quality of digestion, energy absorption and elimination (bowel movement).

Using a food blender analogy, our priority and focus is placed on how well the blender works rather than what is being put into it. Some of the key signs that the blender is not working so well include:

* **Lacking appetite** in the morning
* **Bloating and fatigue** after meals

* **Irritable bowel** in response to certain foods
* **Sugar cravings**.

On the other hand, the most telling signs that the 'blender' is in very good shape is the quality and consistency of the end product i.e. our poo!

There is a lot of information available online about this subject. For example, you can Google and view the famous 'Bristol Chart', to better understand what your stool shape is telling you about your digestive health.

As a Chinese Medicine practitioner I consider the following as signs of healthy bowel movement:

a) **Regular bowel movement**; ideally at least once a day but for some people this could mean twice or three times a day or even once every other day - all of which are fine as long as points b and c below are ticked.

b) **After the job is done, you feel light**, empty and satisfied rather than drained or feeling that you still have more left over.

c) Smooth, well-formed and slightly curved stool that is not sticky (i.e. flushes easily) and that is an even light brown shade.

If your bowel movement does not conform to all or any of the above, there is a good chance that you have some issues with your digestive health. What follows are some general guidelines that can help you get that 'blender' working perfectly again!

1. Eat Warm

If we look at our stomach as a cooking pan, then the nutrition our body gets from food can be likened to the steam that rises from the pan during cooking. If the pan is not warm enough, the foods we eat produce less steam (energy), no matter how nutritious it is.

In Chinese tradition, a sluggish digestion and related symptoms of bloating, indigestion, constipation, diarrhea and so on - can stem from the core problem of a cold pan i.e. weak stomach.

Therefore, we should try to keep the pan hot -i.e. stomach/core temperature warm- to revive sluggish digestion and its associated symptoms.

Here are a few commonly used steps for keeping the 'pan hot' and reviving digestive health:

a) Eat more well-cooked food. Simple and slow cooked stews and soups are easier to digest than salads and cold dishes; because your body has less work to do in breaking the food down into nutrients (i.e. for the pan to create steam). This is why when you are feeling weak, ill or even emotionally unstable your body and stomach's natural healing instincts yearn for simple and warm 'comfort food.'

b) If you prefer to eat cold raw dishes, make sure to balance this with hot meals also. It is true that some foods have highest nutritional value in their raw form and so we must acknowledge that eating some raw food can be beneficial (particularly if you do not have a sluggish digestion). However, if you eat a lot of raw food by itself, this will eventually decrease your core temperature and make it difficult to digest and absorb food.

This is why combining raw dishes with hot foods (soup, tea, and wine) has commonly been practiced in the East for centuries. For example, in Japanese cuisine, a typical meal combines raw and cold sushi with hot Wasabi and Miso soup and heated Sake (rice wine).

c) Do not have a cold drink during or right after meals. This solidifies the oily stuff you have just eaten, making the absorption more difficult. This is why in many restaurants in China, you are commonly served with a pot of hot water or tea before and during your meal.

2. Eat Balanced & Regularly

In gardening, a young plant needs to receive a balanced and consistent intake of water and sunlight to enjoy optimal growth. Too much, too little or sporadic watering or sunlight will damage the plant. Similarly, too much, too little or inconsistent eating patterns can damage our stomach. Below is a brief outline of the kind of care and balance you can provide your digestive system to help it regain full strength:

a) Eat at regular mealtimes: respect the body's natural rhythm by not skipping meals. Wake up the digestive tract with a substantial breakfast. If you skip breakfast you will be more likely to lack appetite at lunch because your digestive tract will not have been awakened. As a result, the body will operate on virtually no energy and go into craving mode especially for sugar - because of low blood sugar levels caused by lack of food later in the afternoon and during dinner time. This can lead to excessive eating and the rise of famine and feasting. It is therefore important to follow a substantial breakfast with a well sized lunch and small simple dinner that allows the stomach to be empty by bedtime.

b) Eat moderate and balanced quantities, avoiding famine and feasting. A traditional Chinese saying advises that we should eat until we are about 80 percent full. This particularly applies to dinnertime because it ensures the stomach is empty by the time you go to bed. Meanwhile, we should be aware of falling into the trap of eating only and too much 'healthy' food. For example, most fruits are good for our health, however consuming them excessively overloads and weakens the stomach; balance is the key.

3. Eat Mindfully

'Eat without a word (conversation)' advised Confucius 2000 years ago. This ancient Chinese teaching is rooted in logical reasoning - because when we are distracted whilst eating we are not chewing well. This overloads our stomach and digestive process with more work to break the food down. We are also more likely to overeat when distracted. Overtime this overloading can contribute to sluggish digestion.

Eating mindfully means being fully focused on eating and feeling your body, your breath and the taste of your food as you eat. This includes chewing your food well (at least 40 times is the commonly recommended amount) until it is almost liquefied. This not only enhances your enjoyment of the food but assists the digestive process -allowing you to get optimal nutritional value out of your meal. It also helps to improve your digestive strength over time.

Today, eating mindfully is not only a matter of not speaking whilst we eat, but also refraining from other distractions such as watching TV or checking our phones and tablets during mealtimes. I recognize that some may find this- especially not speaking at mealtimes-as impractical and out of touch with modern times. My simple view is that if you are serious about returning an already dysfunctional digestive system to full health - you should give this a go.

Otherwise, you can still use the advice offered here as a reminder to tune into your body, your breathing, the taste of the food and chewing - as often as possible when you eat and during any conversations you have as you eat.

Finally, I would advise that you watch the state of mind you eat your meals in. If you eat when angry, worried or very upset (in which case the stomach will be tense) then your digestive system is less capable of doing its work effectively. So try to be in a positive mood when you are eating and don't eat if you are feeling any kind of emotional unease.

4. Eat Sequentially

If you suffer from a weak and problematic digestive system, paying attention to sequential eating (choosing the order you eat various foods) and good food combination (choosing which foods you eat at the same time) may be another useful tool. However, people with an already strong digestive system may not find this advice necessary.

The simple logic is that different foods are not all digested at the same time and rate. Liquids, fruits, vegetables, proteins and carbohydrates are broken down at different rates in the stomach; liquids and fruits being the fastest and proteins and carbohydrates the slowest.

For example, if you eat one meal that combines protein with carbohydrate and also vegetables, then the carbohydrate and vegetables have to effectively sit and wait in line in the stomach while the protein is broken down, causing bloating and indigestion. Similarly, you shouldn't eat fruit after a heavy meal because it will ferment in your stomach as it waits for the other more complex foods to be digested, leading to bloating and gas. If a weak stomach is regularly overloaded and strained in this way it could lead to more problems such as irritable bowel, indigestion and bad poo!

Try to therefore keep your meals as simple as possible so that you are not always eating complex proteins and carbohydrates at the same time; instead you can try either with just vegetables instead. Also remember that fruits should be eaten on an empty stomach for maximum benefit.

Try to experiment with these suggestions to see if it makes a difference to how you feel after meals. There is a lot of online resources about sequential eating and food combination if you are interested to learn more.

Acupuncture for Digesting Well

Over the years, I've used acupuncture to help with a wide range of digestive issues ranging from: reflux, nausea and vomiting to Irritable Bowel Syndrome (IBS), Ulcerative Colitis and Crohn's Disease.

The following is how digestive issue are aided by acupuncture:

* Relieves underlying emotional issues that trigger digestive flare ups (see Chapter 4).

* Improves blood and energy flow to stomach (i.e. helping to heat the pan) - allowing for natural healing and better break down of food.

Chapter 3. Exercise Well

Breathing and Moving well

By speaking of exercising well I'm actually trying to promote good breathing and movement. I define good breathing as being slow and abdominal and good movement as gently working a wide range of muscles and organs without repetitive strain. Why are breath and movement so important when looking at fatigue?

In Chinese medicine, breathing is seen as the primary source for generating and recharging our vital life energy (Qi). The strong and free movement of this energy around the body is also seen by Chinese medicine as instrumental to good health. In fact, the main aim of Chinese medicine practices such as acupuncture, cupping and scraping is to increase the level of energy in the body and or promote its movement where it may be stuck.

This is why exercises that can promote good breathing and movement are so important - especially for those who are fatigued and have no extra energy to burn off.

Introducing Yin Exercises

The right type of exercises for energy recovery are 'Yin' exercises that gently restore, relax, and recharge your body through good breathing and movement.

The ancient Chinese concept of Yin and Yang plays a fundamental role in Traditional Chinese Medicine, and is represented by the famous Yin Yang symbol. In simple terms, Yin and Yang represent the two separate yet opposing energies and sides of all things that together form a whole: for example, mountains and valleys, male and female, sunlight and shade, and cold and hot.

Yin is considered as feminine, cool, soft, dark, and passive. Yang is considered as masculine, hot, hard, light, and active. In the field of sports, Yin exercises are those that are slow and methodical and Yang exercises are those that are fast and forceful. Table 2 over the page provides a general outline of the differences between

Yin and Yang exercises and the following are the general characteristics that define Yin exercises:

a) Deep, soft abdominal breathing. A low intensity exercise that does not leave you out of breath during or after.

b) Gentle and wide range of movement and stretching of the body without repetitive strain on a limited muscle group.

c) Leaves your body (especially hands and feet) warm and energized within but not overly sweaty and fatigued.

Table 2: Yin & Yang Exercises

	YIN	YANG
Typical Exercises	Tai Chi, Qi Gong Yoga Pilates	Weight Lifting Cycling Running
Focus	Internal Goal-less	External Goal-oriented
Effect	Calming Recharging	Exciting Energizing
Characteristics	Slow, Methodical	Fast, Forceful
Develops	-Mind-body coordination, -Mindfulness Relaxation	-Muscle mass, -Physical Strength -Stamina
Disadvantage	Limited physical challenges	Increasing risks of injury & burnout

Some people may find Yin exercises boring and hard to stay in the slow pace. In fact, that is precisely the goal of such exercises; to use gentle and focused movements to force the racing mind to slow down, just like putting the brakes on an over-speeding car.

When people shift their training from Yang to Yin, they may initially feel more fatigued and emotionally flat, because they are suddenly denied of the normal stimuli of adrenaline and endorphins. However, they will find that they can cope better with any such discomforts because their mind has slowed down and become more patient. In the long run, they will normally enjoy greater relaxation, sleep and energy.

Some also worry that they will gain weight without strenuous exercise to burn calories. It is true that most Yin exercises are not designed for weight loss, but for restoration and relaxation. But, as weight gain is usually related to stress, fatigue and digestive issues, it is not uncommon for those who take up relaxing and restorative Yin exercises to see improvements with digestion and weight issues.

Here are the top three Yin exercises I recommend to restore energy:

1. **Tai Chi & Qi Gong**: focuses on one movement flowing into the next slowly and gracefully.

2. **Yoga**: focuses on breathing and stretching. Avoid hot yoga or challenging poses (Asanas).

3. **Pilates**: focuses on breathing and holding and developing core muscles.

There are also some gentle Yang exercises that can -if practiced with a goal-less approach- be suitable for energy recharging. A few notable examples include:

1. **Golf**: just swing and walk in the fresh air. Do not compete with yourself or others.

2. **Swimming**: just breathe, stroke, and glide through the water. Do not count laps. Do not pay attention to technique or speed.

3. **Walking/light jogging**: just find and maintain an easy pace; avoid fatigue.

4. **Cycling**: just pedal at an easy pace and feel the wind on your face. Pay no attention to speed, heart rate or distances.

To recap, the focus on Yin exercises is to guide fatigued people who need to recharge. There are many 'Yang' exercises that have great health benefits - but only for those who have adequate energy levels.

It is all about striking the right balance. Remember that 'Yin Yang' is about wholeness; so we should aim to be fully recharged and able to enjoy a balance of Yin and Yang exercises.

Acupuncture for Exercising Well

Acupuncture compliments exercising well in two ways. One is by treating sprains or strains from Yang exercises (competitive sports or repetitive exercises) allowing you to move well again. The other is by reducing tension in the body and allowing you to breathe better. It does this by helping to:

* Suppress inflammation,
* Increase and enhance blood flow and circulation,
* Reduce tension in the body; especially areas critical to breathing including: upper chest muscles, diaphragm.

Chapter 4. Emotional Wellbeing

Experiencing a wide range of positive and negative emotions is part of a normal life and what makes us whole (keep in mind the Yin Yang theory!).

However, if we frequently experience extremes in emotion such as anger and fear it is likely that we are experiencing some form of emotional imbalance. These imbalances are rooted in what I call the 'emotional container' problem.

Everyone effectively has an emotional container in which we store unwanted emotions such as anger, fear, shame, and anxiety. Shouting when angry, crying when sad, and shaking when afraid are natural reactions that lead to a healthy release of negative emotions. Children are generally so at ease because they are constantly feeling and releasing their emotions freely.

By adulthood we start to reject and repress our emotions. Repressed negative emotions don't just go away, but pile up in our emotional container - which we place a lid on and ignore.

Most of us are doing this to some extent and can live a normal and healthy life doing it for a while. However, if the repression is very frequent and not balanced with healthy expression, the container starts to fill. As it becomes more full we will begin to see some early signs of the building pressure in the form of a restless mind and inexplicable loss of energy and enthusiasm for life (See Table 3).

If we continue stuffing unwanted emotions away and keeping the lid firmly shut the pressure in our container builds so much that the smallest trigger, then sets off an eruption. The usual forms of eruption are also shown in Table 3 over the page.

Table 3. Emotional Container Warning Signs

PRESSURE BUILD UP	ERUPTION
Frequent and underlying feeling of frustration	Uncontrollable angry outburst & rage at relatively minor trigger e.g. road rage
General underlying feeling of anxiety	Panic/Anxiety Attack
Mood Swings & Easily Overwhelmed	Nervous Breakdown
Restless Mind & Poor Sleep Quality	Insomnia
Loss of Enthusiasm & Low Sex Drive	Strong Cravings & Addictions
Regular minor physical ailments i.e. cold and flu, digestive complaints	Flare up of serious illness or disease

These patterns of eruption can be particularly unhealthy if we control and repress the outpouring emotions and physical warning signs again i.e. sweep them back in the container and force the lid shut even harder (including frequent use of medication to quickly suppress any physical signs). This vicious cycle eventually leads to chronic fatigue and illness (i.e. Stages 4-5 from Table 1).

For women, there is a natural process - the menstrual cycle- in which hormonal changes loosens the lid from the emotional container allowing for a regular release of emotional baggage. This release can result in emotional sensitivity or mood swings - but may not be as intense as the eruptions mentioned in Table 3.

Sadly, this healthy and natural process is negatively labeled -Pre-menstrual Tension- so many women do not embrace the emotional releases associated with it; instead, they also can get trapped in the same viscous cycle of release and repression.

So how can we fix this emotional container problem? There are four steps I ask my patients to follow:

1. **Separation and Detachment**
2. **Acceptance**
3. **Harmless Release**
4. **Cultivate Positive Emotions**

Let's look at each of the above in a little more detail.

1. Separation and Detachment

First, we must practice observing our emotions, which are like the currents of a fast flowing river. Our consciousness is often caught up in the river and its endless currents of emotion.

We need to step out of the water and observe the flow of water (i.e. our emotions) from the river bank. This separation and detachment can then help us deal with our 'emotional container' problem. I use the below method to help patients create detachment from emotions (See Appendix 2 for details).

* Mindful Meditation

2. Acceptance:

We have to learn not to judge or resist the feelings we observe because that would just keep us attached to them and give them power to overwhelm us.

Just like treating a child in a tantrum, the more you try to forcefully stop or ignore them, the louder the child becomes. A wise parent lovingly acknowledges the child in their tantrum and gives them time and space to release their frustration; watching them attentively and making sure they are safe without interfering to try and stop it. Once the pressure is released, the child returns to normal.

That is what we can do to deal with our negative emotions or thoughts. Just watch them attentively without trying to stop them. I use the below method to help people accept emotions (see Appendix 3 for details):

* Emotional Freedom Technique (EFT)

3. Harmless Release

Emotions are like a loaded gun. If we fire in the street it is a crime. If we fire on a shooting range, it is a healthy exercise. As far as it disturbs no one, we can release emotions harmlessly. Fear and anger are the most common emotions people suffer. I use the below three methods to help people release fear and anger harmlessly (see Appendix 4 for details):

* Warrior's Breathe
* Trauma Releasing Exercise (TRE)

4. Develop Positive Emotions

According to Yin Yang theory, negative emotions belong to Yin and positive emotions belong to Yang. If we view these emotions as a garden containing Yin and Yang plants, then during the fatigued state the negative emotions have simply outgrown the positive. Once we observe and accept this, we can begin to cultivate the growth of Yang plants (positive emotions) to create balance in the garden.

I have integrated knowledge from positive psychology to offer the below two methods to help people develop positive emotions and enhance their emotional balance and resilience. (See Appendix 5 for details):

* Gratitude Journaling
* Loving-kindness Meditation

Acupuncture for Emotional Well Being

I commonly see strong emotional releases and even healing during or after patient's acupuncture treatments. As the mind and body are strongly connected - areas of tension or pain in the body can sometimes correspond with suppressed emotions or traumas. Acupuncture unlocks these pains and effectively pricks a hole in the emotional container - leading to a release of emotion and pressure. This is aided by:

* Release of endorphins that calm and relax a restless and anxious mind.

*Release of serotonin that can help with those in depressed/low mood.

Remember the emotional release is usually brief and is a part of the healing/detox process. Embrace these changes using the detachment and acceptance methods mentioned earlier so you can let go of the emotion once and for all!

CLOSING REMARKS

I hope you have found this book or at least some of its advice useful. Please remember that energy depletion is a very normal condition of modern day life.

My intention in this book has been to raise your awareness to the signs of fatigue - as they are often overlooked and misunderstood.

I've tried to show you that the solution to rebooting and recharging your body simply lies in natural steps with your sleep, eating, exercise and emotions.

The process of depleting your energy levels and damaging your health often takes years of inadequate rest, poor diet, lack of good exercise and high stress levels. The good news is that reversing the process and regaining full energy and vitality takes a much shorter amount of time (a few months)! You just need to be good to yourself and commit to the simple steps and habits I've covered, that are all in line with the laws of nature.

I wish you all the best on your journey back to full energy and wellbeing!

Qiang Chen

Appendix 1. Guide to Choosing an Acupuncturist

I understand that finding and trying an acupuncturist that you can trust to provide the right results may be a little daunting. I therefore offer the following advice and 3 key steps to help you with the process:

1 - ASK

* Ask friends, family or social media platforms if anyone can recommend an acupuncturist they have personally used.

2 - CHECK

* Once you have shortlisted a few recommended acupuncturists in your area - check their credentials and qualifications:

* In most countries, acupuncturists are qualified by University level degrees and self regulated national registration bodies (e.g. CMBA in Australia, NCCAOM in the USA and BAC in the UK). Find this out from the

practitioner's website or call their office to check their qualification and if they are registered with a national board and associations.

* Most acupuncturists are well rounded practitioners able to deal with a very wide variety of issues. Yet some also get specialised training in various fields such as fertility, psycho-emotional health, sports injuries and so on. If you have a more serious and specific need it is worth refining your search to ask and check for specialised training too; this information should normally be found on the practitioner's websites.

3 - TRY IT

* Once you have selected a suitable acupuncturist - schedule an appointment.

* Ultimately the most important test is how you feel instinctively and connect with the practitioner. Their qualifications or even name/fame is not as important as your gut feeling and the level of care, and attention they pay you when you are with them.

* A good acupuncturist should not rush through the session (with a view to more patients and sales of

services and products). Particularly in the first encounter, they will need to speak to you/get to know you and ask a series of questions about your overall health and lifestyle to better understand your problem and its root causes.

* A good acupuncturist should make you feel safe and comfortable with the advice and treatment they offer you.

Appendix 2. Separation & Detachment

Mindful Meditation

Make sure you sitting or lying comfortably and in a place you know you will not be disturbed for at least 10 minutes and try the following:

1) Close your eyes and take a comfortable deep breath. Then return to just breathing normally.

2) Focus on the feeling of the air gently moving in and out of your nostrils and into your lungs as you breath normally.

3) If any thoughts or feelings or bodily sensations come and distract you -simply notice them without resistance or judgment and return to watching your breath.

4) If you see yourself making any judgment about the thought or feeling or anything else simply notice this

and with every exhalation say "I accept and let go of this judgment."

5) Gently return to watching and feeling your breath.

* Try this for 10-15 minutes every day.

The above is just one very simple method I have developed to help you start detaching from your thoughts and feelings.

These days there are many books and online resources on mindfulness that you can explore. My favourite online resources include:

a. The Great Good Science Center
   http://greatergood.berkeley.edu/topic/mindfulness

b. Mindful Magazine
   http://www.mindful.org/

Appendix 3. Acceptance

Emotional Freedom Technique (EFT)

EFT is a form of psychological acupressure which I have routinely used in my practice for helping my patients accept and release a wide range of emotional issues. It uses tapping with the fingertips on acupuncture points whilst repeating positive affirmations out loud. This clears the "short-circuit" - that has caused the emotional block.

This method is an easy self-help tool to learn and apply. There are plenty good video clips teaching this technique online. My favourite online resource:

a. The official EFT website
    http://www.emofree.com/

b. Dr. Mercola EFT website
    http://eft.mercola.com/

APPENDIX 4: ANGER AND FEAR RELEASE

1. Warrior's Breathe for Anger Release

Find a room where you feel safe and know you will not be disturbed for at least 10 minutes and try the following:

1) Sit comfortably and lean your body forward slightly.

2) Project the person or the event that has made you angry on the wall in front of you and allow the anger to arise.

3) Take a breath as deeply as you can manage.

4) When breathing out, do two things together: Open your mouth and eyes as wide as you can; and breathing out in short bursts making a heavy and strong "HAH" sound from your belly.

5) Repeat the above process three to five times.

6) Watch the anger you have experienced deflate and the body become more relaxed.

This is a method I have developed and that has shown very good results with my patients. Checkout the video demonstration from me at www.chenqiang.net.

You can find many more methods for anger release online. The key is responsible expression & releasing rather suppression!

2. Trauma Release Exercise (TRE) For Fear/Anxiety Release

When we feel fear -we instinctively tense up and curl down slightly to protect our core. To let go of any fear and anxiety or stress that has been repressed in the body I use the Trauma Release Exercise (TRE). TRE induces and uses the body's innate process of involuntary shaking to release suppressed tension and fear in a safe and controlled way.

www.traumaprevention.com is the primary resource for you to learn more about it before giving it a go. You can also find many practical video demonstrations to further guide you online.

Appendix 5: Cultivate Positive Emotions

1. Gratitude Journaling

Keeping a 'gratitude journal' - to write down the things we are grateful for is one of the most popular practices in the field of positive psychology. Researchers have found a wide range of benefits to this practice including improved sleep, increases energy, and enhancing overall satisfaction with life. Gratitude Journaling is particularly powerful when done last thing before bed and/or first thing in the morning.

As an extension to or shorter alternative to the above you can try Three Good Thing (3GT); whereby every night you write down three things that went well that day and their causes.

My favourite resource online is:

a. The Greater Good Science Center:
http://greatergood.berkeley.edu/topic/gratitude

2. Loving-kindness Meditation

Loving-kindness meditation involves extending feelings of compassion toward people, starting with yourself then branching out to someone close to you, then to an acquaintance, then to someone giving you a hard time, then finally to all beings everywhere.

About the Author

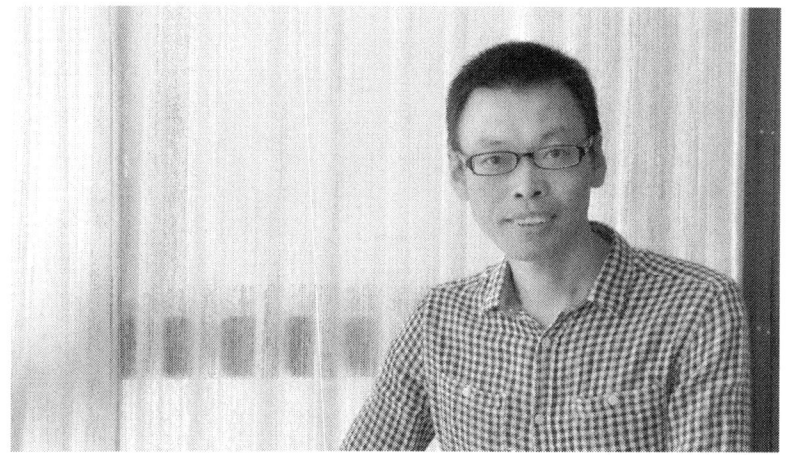

Qiang Chen (Chen) is a National Board registered acupuncturist and Chinese Medicine practitioner in Australia. He established and developed many thriving acupuncture practices in China, United Arab Emirates and Australia during last two decades.

Chen is also the author of two self-help books. He is passionate about empowering others to optimise their body's self-healing mechanism by writing books and teaching online courses.

Chen taught Tai Chi and Qi Gong to diverse audiences since 1997. He gave Chinese Medicine presentations at international conferences and health seminars, medical colleges, hospitals and also at social and supporting groups.

Currently, Chen and his wife live in Canberra. They have one son - a college junior and one cat – who thinks and acts like a dog.

ONE LAST THING...

If you enjoyed this book or found it useful I'd be very grateful if you'd post a short review on Amazon. Your support really does make a difference and I read all the reviews personally so I can get your feedback and make this book even better.

Thanks again for your support!

Printed in Poland
by Amazon Fulfillment
Poland Sp. z o.o., Wrocław